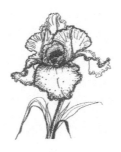

Owings & Rush

The Clitoris Unveiled

The Clitoris Unveiled

Owings & Rush

The Clitoris Unveiled

"Look deep into nature, and then you will understand everything better."

Albert Einstein

Owings & Rush

The Clitoris Unveiled

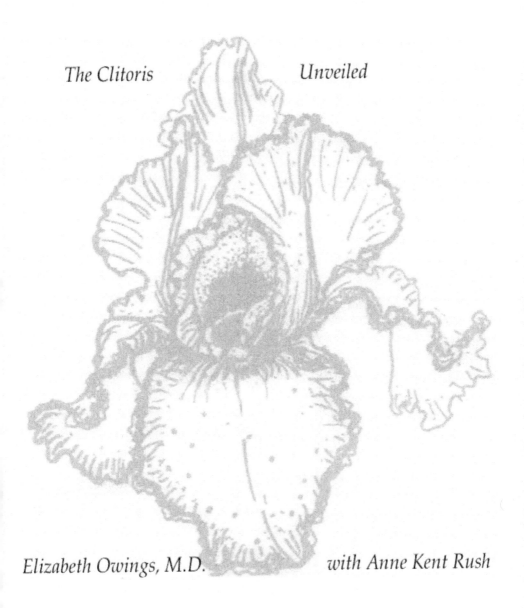

Elizabeth Owings, M.D. with Anne Kent Rush

Orchid Press

Owings & Rush

Text ©Copyright, Elizabeth Owings, MD, January 2019

Illustration & Design ©Copyright, Anne Kent Rush, January 2019

All Rights Reserved. No part of this book may be reproduced or transmitted in any form, electronic or mechanical, including photocopying, recording or by any information storage and retrieval system, without prior written permission of the author and the illustrator. Thank you.

Elizabeth Owings, MD: www.drowingshealth.com

Anne Kent Rush: www.annekentrush.com

ORCHID PRESS
Owings & Rush
P.O. Box 2498,
Daphne, Alabama
36526 USA

TCU-12

First Edition, January 2019
Second Edition, February 14th, 2019
Third Edition July 2020

Library of Congress Cataloging in Publication Number

ISBN 9781795825566

The Clitoris Unveiled

This book is dedicated to

all women and to every person who

compassionately cares for them.

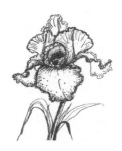

Owings & Rush

THE CLITORIS UNVEILED

CONTENTS

OPENING NOTE
Charles Runels, M.D.- Page 15

SECTION ONE: Secrets & Revelations
The Unveiling – Page 19
Myth vs. Science: The Clitoris – Page 21
Myth vs. Science: Sexual Differentiation – Page 31
In the Beginning – Page 34
Ways We Are All (Comfortingly) Alike
& (Stimulatingly) Different – Page 36

SECTION TWO: Sex-Related Conditions & Treatments
A Doctor Heals Herself – Page 43
Platelet-Rich Plasma (PRP) – Page 44
The O-Shot and The Anatomy of the Clitoris – Page 46
The O-Shot and Urinary Incontinence – Page 49
The Hidden Clitoris – Page 51
Applications for Male Anatomy – Page 52
The P-Shot – Page 52
Pulse Wave Therapy – Page 52
POSTSCRIPT: Back to the Beginning – Page 55

REFERENCES
The Author: Elizabeth Owings, MD – Page 59
Author/Illustrator: Anne Kent Rush – Page 60
Glossary – Page 63
Medical Articles – Page 69
Anatomy Charts – Page 73

Owings & Rush

"The evolution of the field study of female anatomy across the 20th century occurred as a result of active deletion rather than simple omission…. To a major extent its study has been dominated by social factors."

ANATOMY OF THE CLITORIS: HELEN E. O'CONNELL, KALAVAMPARA V. SANJEEVAN AND JOHN M. HUTSON; THE JOURNAL OF UROLOGY, 2005, AMERICAN UROLOGICAL ASSOCIATION

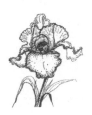

Owings & Rush

OPENING NOTE

For years, the anatomy books did not include the clitoris. Nothing. It was just left out. I have yet to meet a physician who received in medical school detailed instructions on how to examine the clitoris. In my office, I will often examine a woman who suffered with serious disease of the clitoris for many years; but whose gynecologist, in the process of doing routine pap smears, never noticed. That bothers me.

It also bothered Dr. Elizabeth Owings. About six months after I demonstrated for Dr. Owings how to perform the O-Shot® procedure, and after she saw how well it worked to improve the lives of most of the women who received it, she showed up at one of my workshops with a large stack of research papers - everything she could find in the medical literature in one big binder - and presented to the class of physicians the most anatomically and histologically enlightening, and the most beautiful lecture on the clitoris and surrounding tissue that I had ever seen.

I immediately told her, "Every physician and every woman NEEDS to know what you just said. Also, I know the perfect woman to collaborate with you to turn your research and your lecture into a gorgeous, practical book. Physicians can access much material about the penis, but we need something more about the clitoris."

I introduced Dr. Owings to Anne Kent Rush, who has authored and illustrated books on natural healing for over forty years. The result, in your hands now, is a scientific and much needed instructional tool. Moreover, it's a visual and verbal artistic tribute to the amazing and wonderfully made (but too long ignored) special tissue of the female body—the clitoris.

Read and contemplate the beauty and the function of the clitoris; then share the book with your daughter, your doctor, your lover. As a result, the world will become a place with less dis-ease, more understanding and deeper love.

Charles Runels, MD
Inventor of the
O-Shot® Procedure
January 2019

SECTION ONE

Secrets and Revelations

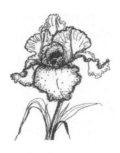

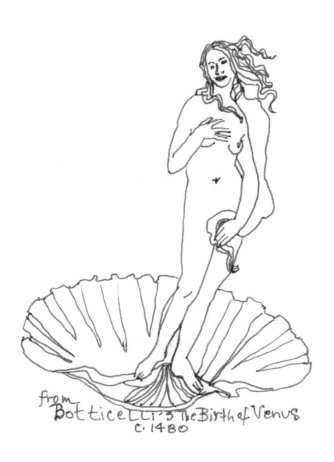

from Botticelli's The Birth of Venus
c. 1480

THE UNVEILING

This is not an encyclopedia with all the answers; that will take years of research to compile. This is a distillation of current scientific facts about the Clitoris System that have been distorted or ignored and need to become known and employed correctly in practical medicine for the health of patients and the peace of mind of their families. From these key guideposts, it is hoped that you will be inspired to engage in your own research to unveil further scientific secrets of the Clitoris.

Enjoy the unveiling!

Elizabeth Owings, M.D. & Anne Kent Rush

Owings & Rush

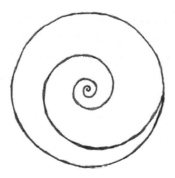

Myth vs. Science: The Clitoris

Myth
Often described as "button-like", the Clitoris is an approximately ½-inch-round, external, female organ (resting above the Urethra) whose function is debatable.

Science
The external "button" of the Clitoris is merely the tip of the internal, 5-to-6-inch-long, nerve-filled, multi-faceted Clitoral organ. The sensitive tip is, however, "button-like", in that its stimulation "turns on" the organ's function: to conduct intense erotic pleasure throughout the internal areas of the Clitoris and further into connected tissues of the woman's pelvis. It is the only system in the human body whose sole function is to produce pleasure.

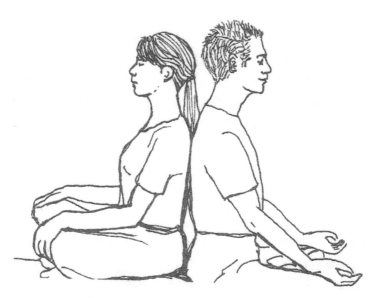
Tantra Back-to-Back Meditation

Myth
The Clitoris System is unique to women in both structure and function.

Science
The Clitoris and male genitals have many identical structures and functions, along with several fascinating differences.

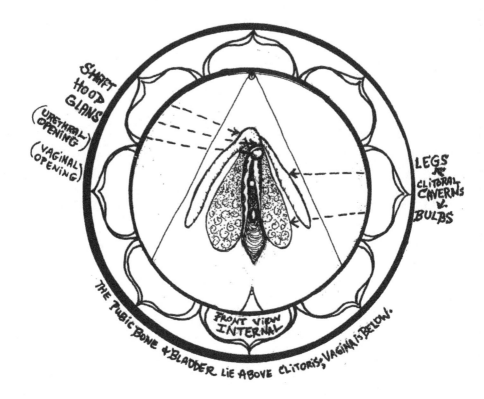

Internal View of Clitoris

Myth
Most well-known medical books contain accurate diagrams of the anatomy of the Clitoris System for reference.

Science
It is almost impossible to find accurate, complete diagrams of the anatomy of the Clitoris System in medical textbooks, vintage or current.

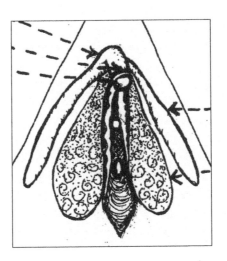

Internal Front View of Clitoris

*"Accurate anatomical information about female pelvic structures should be found in classics, such as Gray's Anatomy, the Hinman urological atlas, sexuality texts such as the classic Masters and Johnson **Human Sexual Response** or any standard gynecologic text. These texts should provide the surgeon with information about how to preserve the innervation and vasculature to the clitoris and related structures, but detailed information is lacking in each of these sources."*

ANATOMY OF THE CLITORIS; HELEN E. O'CONNELL, KALAVAMPARA V. SANJEEVAN, & JOHN M. HUTSON; THE JOURNAL OF UROLOGY, 2005, AMERICAN UROLOGICAL ASSOCIATION

Myth
The Clitoris is a minor, expendable organ with little influence on other body systems.

Science
Because nerves, ligaments and tissue extend from the Clitoris System to all the major, surrounding, pelvic organs, accurate knowledge of the Clitoris System is essential to medical professionals in order to prevent damage to it and to the many inter-connected anatomical structures.

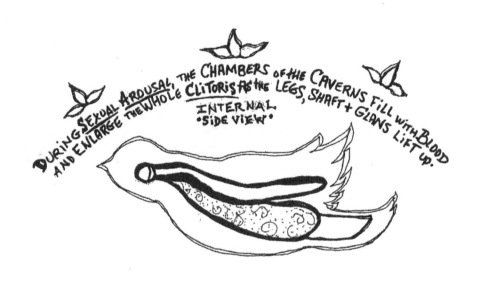
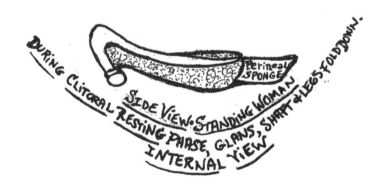

Clitoral Erection

Myth
Only women need to know anything about the Clitoris.

Science
Any medical professionals who treat women patients or any sexual partners of a woman need to understand the basic structure and functions of the Clitoris System if they want to enjoy increasing good health for their patients or heightening erotic stimulation with their partner.

Myth vs. Science: Sex Differentiation

Myth
Human embryos are biologically sex-differentiated at conception.

Science
Human embryos are biologically the same until seven weeks.

Myth
Sex differentiation is triggered in human babies solely by their chromosomes being either combinations of XX (girls) or XY (boys) and is focused in the genitals.

Science
In addition to being influenced by chromosomes, sex differentiation is actually triggered in human babies by the presence or lack of testosterone and the cell receptor for it. Testosterone is stored all over the body, including in brain, muscle, bone, and genitals.

Myth
Chromosome (genetic) sexuality is the same as biological (physical trait) sexuality.

Science
It is possible that a person can have male chromosomes and still develop into a visibly biological female if faulty testosterone receptors change the ability of target cells to respond. Other variations in sexual development that lead to multi-sexual physical and psychological development can occur if dictated by varied combinations of chromosomes, hormones and hormone receptors.

Myth
Mature male and female sexual anatomies are completely different.

Science
Much of female and male genital anatomy is largely the same, appearing different only because female sex organs remain mostly inside the body, while male sex organs emerge to become visible outside the body.

Myth
The Clitoris is a tiny button-like bump located above the Vagina.

Science
The Clitoris consists of a six-inch expansive complex of sensitive structures resting above the Vagina and predominantly inside a woman's pelvis. The button-like bump at the tip of the Clitoral Shaft is analogous to the male penis

head with much the same potential for erotic sensitivity and function of conducting erotic pleasure up the Shaft and into the rest of the pelvis.

Myth
People are either exclusively female or male.

Science
People have subtle combinations of female and male characteristics - detectable now by ever more powerful medical instruments - hormones and their receptors, glands, organs, chemicals and biological features that combine in different proportions to create unique individuals who can decide what gender they prefer to be labeled.

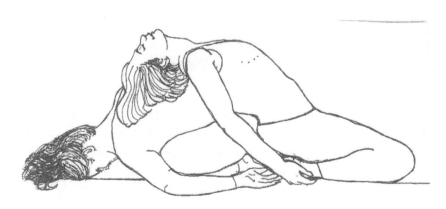

Tantra Yoga Back Rest

In the Beginning

In the beginning is the embryo where all of us begin our existence sharing the same anatomical structure. This underlying anatomical sameness stays with us even after we develop individual sexual characteristics, as gradually, after seven or eight weeks, an embryo begins a process of differentiation.

In most cases, embryos with XY-chromosomes develop full male sexual anatomy, while embryos containing XX-chromosomes develop full female sexual structures. This is true in the majority but not all cases because more biological elements - chromosomes plus hormones and receptors - determine the final details of which exact sex characteristics will manifest in an individual; and there can be a number of variations in the combinations. Testosterone hormone is found in tissues all over the body, including in the brain, and it is the key trigger to sexual differentiation.

Many variations in development can occur depending on the location and amount of testosterone an individual has in different body areas. For example, a person with XY chromosomes (that would in most cases trigger full male body development) may develop breasts and other visibly female body characteristics. In some cases, XY-male chromosome people have a body type of a woman and are voluptuous but do not have a uterus. A person with this combination of features cannot have children but may still look and feel deeply feminine and function happily as a woman in the world.

A key comparative feature of human sexual development is that girls' sex organs remain, for the most part, internal organs, while boys' sex organs emerge from inside the body and establish themselves as external organs.

Another interesting aspect of all human sexual organs, contrary to general social knowledge, is their remarkable functioning similarity. A woman has an internal genital sex organ system, in her pelvis, the Clitoris System that is built and functions in much the same way as the male external, genital organs do - with, of course, several important (and tantalizing) differences.

For many complex social, political and religious reasons, the existence and powerful importance of the female Clitoral System has often been down-played, denigrated or denied at great mental and physical expense to women and the people who love them. Some misogynistic cultures even try to legitimize repression of female pleasure and power by torturing women in the guise of religious ritual and promoting clitoridectomy, that is, surgical removal of the clitoral head, on young girls and women.

The fact, that the Clitoris System is often incorrectly defined and drawn in medical textbooks not only deprives women of accurate knowledge of their bodies for health and pleasure reasons; it also puts women at great risk from medical professionals who may not know the actual facts of female sexual anatomy. Men who love women suffer as well from this lack of anatomical accuracy because they are deprived of facts that could otherwise lead to better informed health decisions and heightened pleasure, intimacy and love between partners.

Ways We Are All (Comfortingly) Alike & (Stimulatingly) Different

A woman's internal **Clitoris System** is homologous, that is, similar in clarifying ways, to the male external genital system in many key aspects.

The small external round mound of the Clitoral Head, or **Glans Clitoris** is often erroneously assumed to be the whole Clitoris. This sensitive spot, appearing above a woman's Vaginal and Urethral openings, is like the head of the external penis in that the Glans is a highly sensitive tip on an extended Shaft. Indeed, if the embryo contained XY chromosomes, it would have become the Glans Penis.

A small strip of skin called the **Clitoral Hood**, which would have become the foreskin or prepuce in a male, covers the body and resting Glans. It recedes when the Clitoral Glans becomes stimulated to expand from increased blood flow during arousal.

The rest of the Clitoris System that corresponds to the male external sex system is internal in women. The internal **Clitoral Shaft** or tube that extends below the Glans head is homologous to the shaft of the penis. Five to six inches long, the nerve-sensitive Clitoral Shaft stiffens and becomes erect when the tip is stimulated, and the shaft takes in more blood as the woman's sexual arousal increases. The Clitoral Shaft is wrapped in spongy Urethral tissue, as is the penis. This spongy tissue wrap in both sexes becomes engorged with blood during stimulation and helps the Shaft to become fuller and erect.

All the tissues in the area can become plush and engorged. Near the Clitoral Shaft and bladder is found the **Grafenberg** or **G-Spot**. The spot is a bit more textured and sensitive when stimulated internally (either through penile intercourse or other means) than its surrounding tissue. One researcher published an article in which he dissected the G-spot eight times. It was usually located on the woman's left, and very near the bladder on the forward side of the vagina. Its forward location may be why some women prefer having their legs upward during intercourse, tilting the pelvis or even being on their stomachs during penile-vaginal intercourse, so that the penis can stimulate it directly.

The Clitoral Shaft has two pairs of side pouches, the **Corpus Cavernosum**, called **Legs** plus the more rounded **Bulbs**. These straddle either side of the Clitoral Shaft and extend below it. The Bulbs are homologous to the spongy tissue surrounding the urethra on the bottom side of the penis. The spongy tissue fills with blood on arousal to stimulate surrounding organs and transmit erotic pleasure.

The O-Spot, a term coined by Charles Runels, M.D., refers to a sensitive area located in the space near the opening of the Vagina, between the Urethra and the Vagina, that is parallel to the internal location of the Skene's Glands. Dr. Runels trains O-Shot® students to inject a person's PRP here because PRP fluid injected in this area can flow from here deeper into the Vaginal, Clitoral and Urethral areas where the PRP can do its most advantageous tissue restoration.

An ejaculatory fluid largely produced in a woman's **Skene's Glands** often is released through the Urethra during sexual excitement, much the way a man's ejaculatory fluids are produced in the testicles and released through the Urethra during arousal and Orgasm. This female release of distinct erotic fluid near or during Orgasm is often mistaken for the excretion of a small amount of urine if the people having sex are not familiar with **Female Ejaculation**.

Dr. Charles Runels is the inventor of the **O-Shot®**, a medical procedure to inject a woman's own PRP (Platelet Rich Plasma) into her vaginal tissue to reduce incontinence and increase orgasmic capability. Dr. Runels chose to place the main injection in the O-Spot area in order to stimulate fluid production in the Skene's Glands as well as rejuvenation of tissues in the surrounding vaginal and urethral tissues. The O-Shot solution to incontinence can be immediate after one quick shot or shortly thereafter and can last for about six months or longer. The quick PRP injection of a person's own blood platelets is safer and more effective than most other more time-consuming, invasive techniques often recommended for stopping incontinence. The O-Shot usually also has the bonus benefit of rejuvenating Vaginal and Urethral tissues to heighten the woman's sexual stimulation and orgasm.

The Glans, Hood, Shaft, Legs and Bulbs connect to form the **Core Clitoris System** whose sole purpose is erotic stimulation.

The Glans, Hood, Shaft, Legs, Bulbs, Urethral Sponge, Skene's Glands and Vagina compose the further aspects of a woman's complex Clitoral System; together they create the **Extended Clitoris System** that heightens and channels erotic stimulation further into the pelvis.

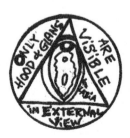

Variations of Sexual Development & Identity

In most cases during the differentiation phase, embryos with XY-chromosomes develop male sexual anatomy, while embryos containing XX-chromosomes develop female sexual structures. This is true in the majority but not all cases because three biological elements – chromosomes, hormones, and hormone receptors - determine the many details of which sex characteristics will manifest in each individual, and there can be a number of variations on the combinations.

Chromosomes determine which genes are expressed, and usually an XX pattern becomes a female and an XY pattern becomes a male. Testosterone, a hormone found in tissues all over the body (including in the brain), strongly influences sexual development, and many variations in sexual development can occur depending on the location, timing, and amount of the exposure.

Some medications given to pregnant women we now know had effects similar to estrogen and testosterone, altering either the appearance of external genitalia or behavior, or both. For example, if testosterone exposure occurs to a developing female embryo, then genitalia which are neither clearly masculine nor feminine may result; it may be a "masculinized" female. Similarly, a male embryo may become "feminized" by hormone or medication exposure. The condition is called "intersex", and modern medicine is still uncovering nuances in the management of these children. The onset of puberty in girls at an ever-younger age and the epidemic of obesity even in children has been attributed in part to the human exposure to estrogens through the hormones given to commercially-raised livestock to fatten them for market.

Hormone receptors play a role in appearance and behavior, as well. A hormone receptor is like the gatekeeper that allows the hormone inside the cell, so it can do its job. For instance, if a person doesn't have normal testosterone receptors, it is possible that a person with XY chromosomes (that would in most cases trigger male sexual development) may develop exterior female characteristics, because the cells are unable to respond to testosterone. This person with male marker chromosomes would have no uterus or complete vagina but still could develop breasts and an otherwise distinctly female body type, and though unable to bear children, feel feminine, appear to be a woman and function that way. This rare condition is called "testicular feminization". A new model for counseling and medically treating biologically trans-gendered patients is needed. Feelings of femininity and masculinity are not "all in our heads"; they are largely rooted in our biology. The details of the testosterone and chromosome interaction in sex development would be crucial to developing nuanced treatments.

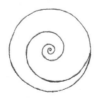

SECTION TWO

Sex-Related Conditions & Treatments

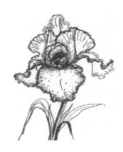

"Anyone who says he can see through women
is missing a lot."

Groucho Marx

Sex-Related Conditions & Treatments

A Doctor Heals Herself
By Elizabeth Owings, MD

I've always had a thirst for knowledge and love of teaching. After medical school, I completed residencies in Pediatrics, General Surgery, and Pediatric Surgery Critical Care. It was during my General Surgery training at Tulane that I received the 'I Mims Gage Teaching Award', presented to the surgery resident who received the highest evaluations from the residents and students—in other words, "from whom did they learn the most?" Through the study of Pediatrics, I learned embryology; through the study of Surgery—which does not always include an operation—I learned physiology and the mechanisms of injury; and through Surgery and Critical care, I gleaned the amazing healing which is possible in the presence of the synergy of operative repair, non-operative support, and nutrition. In short, I have studied how the body forms, performs, and heals itself.

My official training stretched to fourteen post-graduate years, yet my love for learning is so great that I still keep up with my post-graduate calendar as if each year is an official year of training (roughly PGY-30). My practice has ranged from chief medical advisor of a supplement company (further astounding me as to the possibilities of healing when the body is supplied with the necessary materials), to primary care physician, urgent care physician, emergency room physician, and private practice physician in aesthetic and concierge medicine. All told, it's humbling: I may remove the infected appendix or cast the fracture, but who heals the body? Who is responsible for the return of optimal function—*or any function at all?*`

Despite all this expertise, in 2015, at fifty-years old, I found myself overweight, suffering through menopause, occasionally incontinent, deeply depressed – and to seal the misery, unable to have an orgasm at all. My medical colleagues seemed to offer no real solutions. I felt hopeless and ready to die.

Then light came from an unexpected source. A medical equipment representative told me about a promising new procedure, the O-Shot® for improving sexual function with PRP, or Platelet-Rich Plasma, a serum extracted from your own blood to inject into damaged tissues – and the inventor lived just a few hours south. After researching the procedure, I decided to try the O-Shot®. Three weeks to the day after my O-Shot® - that took a few minutes – I had my first orgasm in over a year. To top off that treat, my urinary incontinence ended. These remarkable results marked the beginning of a rejuvenated personal life as well as a fascinating new professional focus devoted to training in and administering healthy healing treatments for a variety of sexual dysfunctions as well as aesthetic issues. I was inspired to spread the joy!

Platelet-Rich Plasma (PRP)

Platelets are the components of blood that tell your body to stop bleeding and start healing after injury. It's possible to isolate this component with a small, tabletop, medical device called a "centrifuge" that can be used in an office or hospital setting. For many years, PRP has been employed in elite athlete care, chronic wound management, dental surgery and veterinary surgery. PRP can improve the function of damaged nerves (even years after the injury), decrease abnormal inflammation, and help heal tissues with poor blood supply, like tendons and ligaments. It has been extensively studied, and there has never been a serious complication through its use. The general consensus for the timing of results from PRP is that the onset of its deep regenerative action comes about three weeks after injection, with full healing effects manifesting in about three months; however, joint pain and some other issues can improve noticeably within a few days.

I was on fire to help as many women as I could so they would experience the benefits I'd had from the O-Shot®. I became certified by the treatment's inventor, Dr. Charles Runels. Then I lined up as many patients as possible for the procedure. My third patient had a condition called Lichen Sclerosus, or Lichen Sclerosus and Atrophy. In this condition, the Clitoris may become completely covered by tissue that scars and grows together. The Vagina becomes dry, and intercourse becomes so painful that it may be impossible. The normal tissues around the Vagina begin to shrink and disappear. As it turns out, PRP can be used for very effective treatment of this condition, but I didn't know that at the time. However, I did realize that I didn't know nearly enough about the anatomy of the areas needing treatment, so I began serious research into relevant articles and medical studies.

The first place online a doctor usually goes to learn about medical questions is a website called PubMed. A simple two-word search for "clitoris" and "anatomy" yields a whopping 1,280 articles, of which about 20 proved quite informative. The clitoris has been completely removed from some versions of anatomy books over the past 200 years. In fact, as far as my medical school anatomy professor was concerned, it was unimportant. However, it is still a topic of interest to serious researchers in the current day.

I spent the next sixty days and about three hundred dollars downloading medical articles about anatomy, and I ran across some fascinating information I share with you in these chapters. From the outset, I didn't assume I already knew everything. Every doctor who attends my lecture says they've learned something or seen an image they had never seen before. Our anatomy professor in medical school dismissively skipped over the topic, telling his students that the clitoris was "just a puny homologue of the penis". "Homologue" means everything you find in one has a similar part on the other. The information on the powerful and unique aspects of the Clitoris that I uncovered and organized puts all misinformed professors' puny myths to rest.

I wanted to re-examine the complete anatomy of all of the sexual structures in women because I realized that though doctors are doing many procedures on these areas, many of the reference anatomy books aren't complete, and some textbooks contain blatant inaccuracies. Fortunately, the study of female genital anatomy is vibrantly alive, and I've been able to learn a great deal from the work of others.

The O-Shot® and the Anatomy of the Clitoris

Once I began looking into the anatomy, I became amazed that, though the penis and clitoris were almost entirely homologous, the anatomical labels they'd been given were completely different.

The only portion of the Clitoris visible externally is the very tip, or Glans; a small portion of the body just above it can be felt but is covered by mucosa and the prepuce. The body is composed of the joined internal tubes similar to the penis in which they are called the Corpora Cavernosa. The Glans of the Clitoris is attached under the moist mucosa of the Vulva to the Bulbs of the Vestibule that are homologous to the corpus spongiosum in the male. Unlike the male element, the Urethra and Vagina are straddled by the divided Bulbs. The legs of the Clitoris travel deep, overlying the tissues of the Bulbs, and lie on either side of the vagina. The deepest portion of the legs to the tip of the Glans Clitoris averages 5.5 inches in length (about 14 cm).

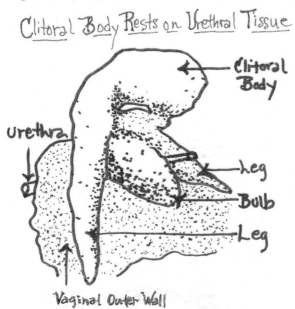

The introduction of PRP into the area with the O-Shot® yields improved sexual response as well as improved urinary continence, vaginal lubrication, and sexual desire. Chronic pain from mesh, episiotomy scars, and abnormal inflammatory states such as Lichen Sclerosus and interstitial cystitis may also be improved (the latter even though no PRP is introduced into the bladder).

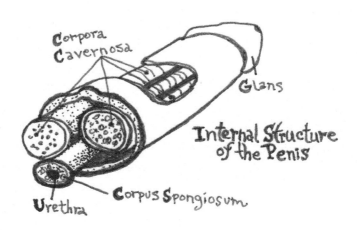

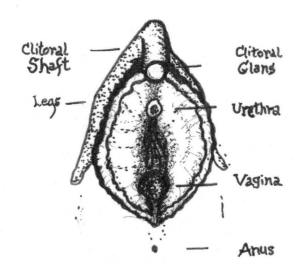

The O-Shot & Urinary Incontinence

Urinary incontinence (UI) is the undesired leakage of urine. There is "stress incontinence" which means we leak urine when we cough or sneeze, and "urge incontinence" which means we leak urine when we have to urinate, and we may not make it to the bathroom in time. It is more common in women than men, but still occurs as a complication to surgery or medical conditions for many men. Urinary incontinence is a massive problem few people talk about. It occurs in 20% of women age 20 and about 50% of women age 50, *whether or not they have ever given birth.* An interesting study of menopausal sisters, one pair of whom had had children and one of whom had not, found very similar incidence of 47% and 49%, with higher likelihood in the sisters of the incontinent women.

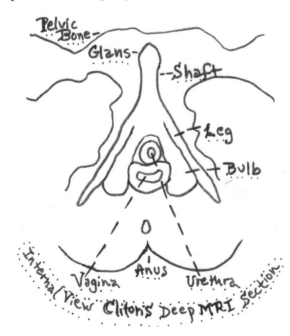

UI is a treatable condition. Some people can do pelvic floor exercises called Kegels, strengthening the muscle responsible for continence. Some can be helped by behavior modification, in which women will empty their bladder more frequently and possibly drink less water than usual. When that doesn't work, they may be placed on medication which may give them side effects of dry mouth and blurry vision. Some are helped by topical estrogen, but this is not an option for every person with incontinence. Urethral inserts, pessaries (rigid ring inserted into the vagina), Botox (for overactive bladder), radiofrequency, and sacral nerve stimulators all have had some success. Surgery is an option many women resort to, with mixed results. Some are cured, while some have painful complications.

Among women who have never had children, factors that increase pressure in the abdomen increase the incidence of UI. Such factors include high BMI, straining due to constipation, high impact exercises, or a high volume of low impact exercises. Sisters of women with UI are at higher risk, as well.

In men, Urinary Continence is due to a circular band of muscle that constricts to stop the flow of urine. In contrast, women's continence is supported by several synergistic structures, four of which are easy to grasp: (1) cavernous erectile tissues overlying the first one-third of the urethra; (2) a thin band of muscle overlying but not encircling the cavernous tissues and the first two-thirds of the urethra; (3) the front wall of the vagina and (4) the legs and bulbs of the Clitoris. Once I understood how delicate the female continence mechanism was, I was amazed that it ever worked correctly.

You might wonder what purpose a clitoral injection serves in treating urinary incontinence? The legs of the Clitoris are close and often touching the urethra. We don't know yet the full benefits of the Clitoral PRP injection. We have noticed in working with PRP that conditions near the injected areas are helped not simply the original injection spots. Many providers who care for women with a condition called interstitial cystitis, or chronic bladder inflammation are helped by the O-Shot®, even though no PRP is placed into the bladder. It's possible that the PRP also gives some support to the muscle. Many providers who use PRP for hair restoration find that areas they did not inject still show benefit. We don't know exactly where the beneficial effects cut off. Does it benefit only the tissue where we injected it, or does it repair nearby tissues as well?

The Hidden Clitoris: Phimosis Lichen Sclerosus and Atrophy

The Journal of Obstetrics and Gynecology from just a couple years ago published an article titled, "Acute presentation of clitoral Phimosis in a 16-year old girl," which is another way of saying she had Lichen Sclerosus - the patient's condition that drove me to read all these articles. Phimosis meant the Clitoral Hood was attached down to the Clitoral Glans and couldn't be pulled away. It probably had been developing in my patient for some months or years. This is a condition that I think is much more common than we realize.

To get an idea of how disfiguring this condition can be, go to your images section of your web browser and type in Lichen Sclerosus. Many of the women afflicted say they don't even feel like women anymore. Being confronted with this is what drove me to search the literature.

Apparently, an autoimmune condition, Lichen Sclerosus is an abnormal inflammatory state in which the tissues of the vulva shrink and disappear. The prepuce adheres tightly to the Glans Clitoris, and the tissues of the Vulva fuse over it so that it may not be seen at all. The Vagina becomes dry and intercourse becomes painful, if it can be accomplished at all. Due to this abnormal inflammation, there is an increased incidence of cancer of the vulva. Medical treatments have been limited to testosterone and anti-inflammatory creams. Newer treatments employing office techniques to release the clitoris and introduce PRP have been quite promising, restoring some women to their pre-lichen health.

Applications for Male Anatomy

The P-Shot® or Priapus Shot®

PRP injections can also be very effective in improving male sexual responses as well as female. One of Dr. Runels' main patented treatments for male sexual issues is called the P-Shot® or Priapus Shot®. It involves a procedure for injecting into the shaft of the penis at several spots as well as into the glans with a patient's own blood-derived growth factors in their Platelet-Rich Plasma. This rejuvenates the tissues and functions of the penis. Within three weeks or less, the PRP helps rejuvenate the blood vessels and tissues in the penis so that blood flow and strength are improved; and the penis is able to become larger and firmer during sexual arousal for longer periods of time. Even men with sexual dysfunction due to surgery and diabetes can see benefits.

This is the same response that the tissues in the Clitoris show after PRP/ O-Shot® injections.

Low-Intensity Shock Wave Therapy: Pulse Wave Therapy

A new technique for treating erectile dysfunction involves applying low-intensity shock wave pulses to the penis and surrounding blood vessels. The vessels are temporarily stretched many times, causing changes in gene expression resulting in new blood vessels to the area. The results take four to twelve weeks but are very promising.

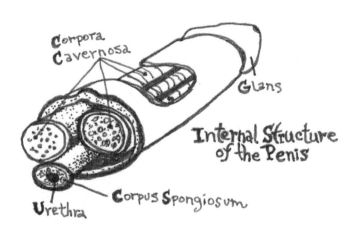
Internal Structure of the Penis

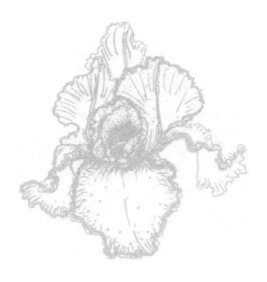

"Nothing in life is to be feared; it is only to be understood.
Now is the time to understand more,
so that we may fear less."

Marie Curie

POSTSCRIPT

For too long, women and men have lived as though idealized unnatural versions of our selves are reality. This habit of divorcing ourselves from nature has confused our thinking and crippled our ability for intimacy and true learning. Medicine has been damaged because many texts and professors are either ignorant or indifferent to the facts of human sexual anatomy because they do not fit into their bias or worldview. How many women have been denied accurate anatomical information or been injured because correct female anatomy had not been taught? Enough! Now's the time to face the facts—they are much more interesting than the myths. We will all benefit from the truth because, in addition to enabling women to know and enjoy their own bodies more, it will set free medical minds to practice more responsible medicine and engage in more useful research. This book is an effort to present hard to find information in an accessible format and stimulate others to pursue more answers about this fascinating aspect of our world.

Enjoy the unveiling!

Owings & Rush

REFERENCES

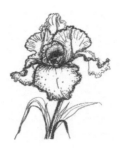

Owings & Rush

ELIZABETH OWINGS, MD

Dr. Elizabeth Owings has a doctorate in medicine from the University of Alabama School of Medicine in Birmingham, Alabama. Her extensive training includes residencies in Pediatrics, Surgery, Critical Care Medicine and Pediatric Surgery. She has served as the Chief Medical Advisor for herb, vitamin and supplement manufacturing companies for several years. Always interested in mechanisms, she used that time to learn how natural products could restore the body to a state of health. Her practice in Fairhope, Alabama centers on general aesthetics as well as men's and women's sexual function. She received the I. Mims Gage Teaching Award from Tulane University in 1994, and has been training and teaching in the southeast in the ensuing decades. She is a certified trainer for the Vampire® procedures, including the O-Shot® and the P-Shot®. Her background in surgery and anatomy makes her uniquely suited to bring you the newest information on female anatomy found in this book.

www.DrOwingsHealth.com

ANNE KENT RUSH

Publications: Rush has published many magazine articles, ghost written four and authored 17 books (including 13 in her specialty field of preventive health care), that have sold millions & been translated into 12 languages.

GETTING CLEAR: Bodywork for Women; Random House, Inc., 1972.
FEMINISM AS THERAPY; Mander & Rush; Random House, Inc., 1974.
MOON, MOON: A History of Moon Mythology; Moon Books/Random House, 1976.
THE BASIC BACK BOOK; Complete Back Care; Summit/Simon & Schuster, 1979.
GRETA BEAR GOES TO YELLOWSTONE NATIONAL PARK; Greta Bear Enterprizes, 1984.
THE BACK RUB BOOK; Vintage Books, 1989.
ROMANTIC MASSAGE; Avon Publishers, 1991.
THE MODERN BOOK OF MASSAGE; Dell Publishers, 1994.
THE MODERN BOOK OF YOGA; Dell, 1996.
THE MODERN BOOK OF STRETCHING; Dell, 1997.
The Omega Book of BODYWORK BASICS; Dell, 2000.
CLASIC CAMEOS & IMCOMPARABLE INTAGLIOS; Jules & Gem Productions, 2K.
MASSAGE FOR TOTAL WELL-BEING; Universe/Rizzoli Publishers, 2001.
THE WAY OF STRETCHING; Little, Brown Publishers, 2005.
WOMEN'S HORMONES; with Charles Runels, MD; LifeStreamMedical, 2009.

CONTEMPORARY SPORT ART; with Tobin Terry; United States Sports Academy, 2010.
THE CLITORIS UNVEILED, Elizabeth Owings, MD with Rush; Orchid Books, 2019.

Graphic Design & Illustration: As well as her own books, Rush has designed & illustrated many projects for clients. The most well-known bestsellers illustrated by Rush are: THE TASSAJARA BREAD BOOK, Ed Brown, Shambhala Publications; and THE MASSAGE BOOK, George Downing, Random House, 1971. Her recent illustrated books are THE LISTENING HAND by Ilana Reubenfeld; Bantam, 2000; and GO SOUTH TO FREEDOM by Frye Gaillard, New South Books, 2017.

Businesses: Rush co-founded the Esalen Institute Women's Studies Department, Big Sur; the Alyssum Women's Therapy Center, San Francisco; and Moon Books Publishers, Berkeley & N.Y. Rush has been a consultant to several firms starting in-house publishing branches, including San Francisco Friends Center and the Oakland Museum of Art. Rush was a partner in the Alabama songwriting team, Amazing Grits Music. Rush has a B.A. in English Composition, Minor in Painting, from Wayne State University, and post degree studies in Etching at the Boston Museum School of Fine Arts. From 2007-2008 Rush designed and wrote marketing material for RIISnet, Inc., an international technology company. Currently Rush has a freelance business to write, edit and design books, marketing material and logos for companies and individuals.

www.AnneKentRush.com

Owings & Rush

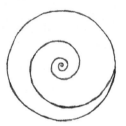

GLOSSARY
CLITORIS-RELATED TERMS

Anus-the opening through which solid waste leaves the body

Bartholin's Glands – Two small external openings on the Vulva to either side of the Vaginal opening lead to these glands that excrete lubricating fluid during a woman's erotic arousal; homologous to male's Cowper's Glands that excrete popularly-named "pre-come" fluid during sexual arousal

Bladder-(urinary bladder)-the organ which stores urine from the kidneys and empties it through the urethra

Blood Vessel-the tubular structure that delivers blood to tissues and returns it to the heart and lungs

Bulbs-(vestibular bulbs)-erectile tissue which overlies the urethra and surrounds the vagina. It is frequently depicted as though within the labia minora, but it is actually quite deep. It is the female homologue of the male corpus spongiosum, the spongy tissue which surrounds the urethra. It is a single midline structure in the male, but is bifid, or split in two in the female.

Circulation-movement of fluid in a closed system, in this case, the movement of blood throughout the body

Clitoris-generally refers to the female external genitalia, homologous to the male penis and glans; internally it is bifid, or split in two connected legs overlying the urethra and straddling the vagina

Clitoris System:
Clitoris System Core: Glans, Hood, Shaft, Legs, Bulbs
Clitoris Extended System: Glans, Hood, Shaft, Legs, Bulbs, Urethra, Skene's Glands, O-Spot®

Clitoridectomy – removal of the external tip of the Clitoral Glans

Corpus Cavernosum, plural corpora cavernosa-the erectile tissue which allows for erections

Corpus Spongiosum- erectile tissue surrounding the urethra in the male, connecting to the glans. The tissue is present in the female, and will become larger and can be dissected out if a woman is given large amounts of testosterone as a precursor to a sex change operation

Ejaculation-the rhythmic, forceful discharge of semen from the penis, usually accompanied by orgasm. It can also occur in females, with fluid from Skene's Glands expelled forcefully through the urethra.

Ejaculatory Fluid – See Skene's Glands.

Erect-engorged with blood and firm, rigidly upright and straight

Erectile Tissue--tissue well-supplied with blood which can become engorged during sexual arousal, leading to erections in men and women

Estrogens-hormones present in both men and women (there are four naturally occurring estrogens). In women, levels rise and fall based on her menstrual cycle; levels are generally stable and lower in children and menopausal women. In men, higher than normal levels can lead to fatigue, weight gain, and loss of libido. The primary source of estrogen in men is from the breakdown product of testosterone.

Female Orgasm System-The Glans, Shaft, Legs, Bulbs, Urethral Sponge and also Vagina compose the major parts of a woman's complex Clitoral System that form the Female Orgasm System.

Glans -The glans penis or glans clitoris refers to the rounded end of the penis or the Clitoris.

G-Spot-refers to an area deep in the vagina which is claimed to yield greater sexual arousal and possibly ejaculation. It is supposed to be just beneath the front wall of the vagina, near where the bladder empties into the urethra. Its presence is still quite controversial, with modern medical journals serving as the forum for open debate between the experts in female anatomy. One university-associated physician claims to have dissected it out and offers pictures and microscopic evidence of a highly vascular nerve bundle. It is either on the left or right, but never midline. Conversely, other university-affiliated physicians have performed extensive dissections and can find no evidence of such a thing, certain the other doctor has merely identified lateral vaginal wall veins. (Go to www.pubmed.gov and enter the term G-spot to get the highlights.) Despite the controversy, many women and their lovers find deep stimulation of the forward wall of the vagina to be a different kind of stimulation than experienced during stimulation of the clitoris or general stimulation of the vagina without isolating this area.

Hood-(clitoral hood)-the female foreskin or prepuce, that covers the glans of the clitoris in the un-aroused state

Hormone-a cellular messenger

Incontinence (UI, urinary incontinence) - the distressing involuntary leakage of urine. It may be "stress incontinence", when during a cough or sneeze or anything which increases pressure inside the abdomen urine leaks out, or "urge incontinence"; when the urge to urinate occurs, the urge is so strong and abrupt the person can't get to the toilet in time.

Labia-Latin for "lips", can refer to the outer lips (labia majora), the inner lips (labia minora) or all of them

Legs of the clitoris - the deep or internal portions of the Clitoris which overlie or straddle the Urethra and lie on each side of the Vagina; also called crura.

Mound of Venus – Mons Pubis - Female center of pelvic bone structure above genitalia, for protection of internal organs and padded with fatty tissue for comfort during sexual pressure

Non-orgasmic-unable to achieve an orgasm by any means, in the presence of sufficient sexual stimulation. **Pre-Orgasmic** is often a preferred term as it indicates the possibility of healing.

Orgasm-climax of the sexual response, experienced as intensely pleasurable peak sensations centered in the genitals

O-Shot®- or Orgasm Shot® is a medical procedure using a woman's own platelet-rich plasma to rejuvenate sexual function and/or urinary continence

Penis-external male organ for sexual expression and urination

Perineum-the external area between the anus and the scrotum in men or Vulva in women

Periurethral Spongy Tissue – Cavernous structures overlying (not surrounding) the Urethra within 15 mm of the Bladder; Appear to function in support of Urinary continence as well as increase of erotic pleasure as they expand on stimulation filling with blood and pressing on surrounding tissues

The P-Shot® - Priapus Shot® – Specialized medical introduction of PRP into the penis

Pubic Bone-where the pelvis joins in front. It is covered by the area which has been called the "root" of the Clitoris, where the clitoral body, legs (or crura) and the vestibular bulbs join. The soft tissues between the pubic bone and vulvar surface have also been called the Urethral Sponge.

Sacrum-the lowest portion of the pelvis in the back, at the base of the spine

Scrotum-the sack which holds the testicles; it hangs away from the body so the testicles remain cool for optimal sperm development.

Shaft-the long portion of something; in the penis, it supports the glans; in the Clitoris, it is covered by the prepuce and ends in the glans Clitoris.

Skene's Glands-female homologue to the male prostate. They empty into the distal urethra and secrete a thick, white fluid with measurable prostate-specific antigen (PSA). See references by Pastor, Rubio, et al.

Sperm-the male reproductive cell

Testosterone-the hormone present in both men and women responsible for "androgenization", or "man-ness", promoting greater bone and muscle density alone, with increased libido. When too much is present in women, they may grow hair on their faces; in men extreme aggression and high blood pressure may result, as well as increased blood 'density', or elevated red blood count.

Urethra-the tube leading from the bladder through which urine is excreted

Urethral Sponge - (periurethral sponge) erectile tissue overlying the urethra on the top and both sides but not all the way around. An internet search of the terms will display diagrams of spongy tissue encircling the urethra, but the literature does not support this notion. See Baggish and O'Connell.

Urine-the liquid waste filtered by the kidney, stored in the urinary bladder and voided from the body via the urethra

Vagina - *internal* female genital canal, popularly named "the Birth Canal", that extends from the Vulva to the Uterus

Vulva - *external* female genitalia, including Labia, Clitoral Glans & Hood, Pubic Mound, Vaginal opening, Bartholin's Glands' openings

Medical Articles

Al-Mukhtar Othman J, Akervall S, Milsom I, Gyhagen M. Am J Obstet Gynecol. 2017 Feb; 216(2):149.e1-149.e11. Epub 2016 Oct 6. **Urinary incontinence in nulliparous women aged 25-64 years: a national survey.**

Almousa S, Bandin van Loon A. Maturitas. 2018 Jan; 107:78-83. Epub 2017 Oct. **The prevalence of urinary incontinence in nulliparous adolescent and middle-aged women and the associated risk factors: A systematic review.**

Alves JO, Luz STD, Brandão S, Da Luz CM, Jorge RN, Da Roza T. Int J Sports Med. 2017 Nov;38(12):936-941. Epub 2017 Sep 26. **Urinary Incontinence in Physically Active Young Women: Prevalence and Related Factors.**

Baggish M, Steele A, Karram M. J Gyn Surg. 15(4). Epub 30 Jan 2009. **The Relationships of the Vestibular Bulb and Corpora Cavernosa to the Female Urethra: A Microanatomic Study Part 2.**

Bardino M, Di Martino M, Ricci E, Parazzini F. J Paediatric Adolescent Gynecol. 2015 Dec; 28(6):462-70. Epub 2015 Jan 7. **Frequency and Determinants of Urinary Incontinence in Adolescent and Young Nulliparous Women.**

Buchsbaum GM, Duecy EE. Neurourol Urodyn. 2008; 27(6):496-8. **Incontinence and pelvic organ prolapse in parous/nulliparous pairs of identical twins.**

Carvalhais A, Natal JR, Bø K. Br J Sports Med. 2018 Dec; 52(24):1586-1590. Epub 2017 Jun 22. **Performing a high-level sport is strongly associated with urinary incontinence in elite athletes: a comparative study of 372 elite female athletes and 372 controls.**

Eliasson K, Larsson T, Mattsson E. Scand J Med Sci Sports. 2002 Apr;12(2):106-10. **Prevalence of stress incontinence in nulliparous elite trampolinists.**

Hoag, N, Keast, J, O'Connell, H. J Sex Med. 2017 Dec; 14(12):1524-1532.**The "G-Spot" Is Not a Structure Evident on Macroscopic Anatomic Dissection of the Vaginal Wall.**

Oakley SH, Mutema GK, Crisp CC, Estanol MV, Kleeman SD, Fellner AN, Pauls RN. J Sex Med. 2013 Sep;10(9):2211-8. Epub 2013 Jun 27. **Innervation and histology of the clitoral-urethral complex: a cross-sectional cadaver study.**

O'Connell HE, DeLancey JO. J Urol. 2005 Jun;173(6):2060-3. **Clitoral anatomy in nulliparous, healthy, premenopausal volunteers using unenhanced magnetic resonance imaging.**

O'Connell HE, Sanjeevan KV, Hutson JM. J Urol. 2005 Oct; 174 (4 Pt 1):1189-95. **Anatomy of the Clitoris.**

Ostrzenski A, Krajewski P, Ganjei-Azar P, Wasiutynski AJ, Scheinberg MN, Tarka S, Fudaleg M. BJOG. 2014 Oct;121(11):1333-9. Epub 2014 Mar 19. **Verfication of the anatomy and newly discovered histology of the G-spot complex.**

Pastor A, Chmel R. Int Urogynecol J. 2018 May;29(5):621-9. Epub 2017 Dec 28. **Differential diagnostics of female "sexual" fluids: a narrative review.**

Rubio-Casallas A, Jannini EA, J Sex Med. 2011 Dec;8(12):3500-4. Epub 2011 Oct13. **New Insights from One Case of Female Ejaculation.**

Tettamanti G, Altman D, Cnattingius S, Bellocco R, Iliadou AN. Int Urogynecol J. 2014 Nov;25(11):1471-7. Epub 2014 May 8. **Does urinary incontinence have fetal origins? Results from a nationwide twin study.**

Tsutsumi S, Kawahara T, Hattori Y, Mochizuki T, Teranishi JI, Makiyama K, Miyoshi Y, Otani M, Uemura H. J Med Case Rep. 2018 Feb 14;12(1):32. **Skene duct adenocarcinoma in a patient with an elevated serum prostate-specific antigen level: a case report.**

Van Turnhout AA, Hage JJ, van Diest PJ. Acta Obstet Gynecol Scand. 1995 Nov;74(10):767-71. **The female corpus spongiosum revisited.**

The following chart shows how female and male genital forms develop matching elements; but because most have been given differing scientific labels, these similarities are obscured and not widely recognized.

Sameness of Human Embryologic Female and Male Genital Forms

Eight-week-old human embryos have identical genital tubercle structures consisting of: glans area, the urogenital groove and fold, and labioscrotal folds. These elements later develop into female and male sex organs with some structural differences yet continued functional similarities. To clarify the dominance of female and male sexual organ similarities over their differences, the following chart delineates the many instances in which female and male sex organs with extremely different given labels mostly retain structural similarities and perform the same biological functions.

<u>Embryologic Precursor becomes:</u>	<u>Female:</u>	<u>Male:</u>
1. Genital Tubercle	**Clitoris:** **Glans Clitoris** **Clitoral Crura** **Vestibular Bulbs**	**Penis:** **Glans Penis** **Corpora Cavernosa** **Corpus Spongiosum**
2. Prepuce	Clitoral Hood	Foreskin

3. Labioscrotal Folds	Labia Majora	Scrotum
4. Urogenital Folds	Labia Minora	Penis Skin
5. Urogenital Sinus	Bartholin's Gland Bladder & Urethra Skene's Glands	Cowper's Gland Bladder & Urethra Prostate
6. Gonad	Ovary Rete Ovarii	Testis Rete Testis

	Female	Male
7. Müllerian or Mesonephric Tubule	Epoophoron or Paroophoron	Paradidymis or Efferent Ducts
8. Mesonephric Duct (Wolffian Duct)	Gartner's Duct	Epididymis Seminal Vesicle Vas Deferens
9. Paramesonephric (Müllerian Duct)	Fallopian tubes Uterus, cervix, vagina	Appendix Testis Prostatic utricle
10. Gubernaculum	Round Ligament of Uterus	Gubernaculum Testis
11. Lateral Perineal Folds	Perineal Body	Perineal Body

Urinary incontinence (UI) is the undesired leakage of urine. There is "stress incontinence" which means we leak urine when we cough or sneeze, and "urge incontinence" which means we leak urine when we have to urinate, and we may not make it to the bathroom in time. It is more common in women than men, but still occurs as a complication to surgery or medical conditions for many men. Urinary incontinence is a massive problem few people talk about. It occurs in 20% of women age 20 and about 50% of women age 50, *whether or not they have ever given birth.*

UI is a treatable condition. Some people can do pelvic floor exercises called Kegels, strengthening the muscle responsible for continence. Some can be helped by behavior modification, in which women will empty their bladder more frequently and possibly drink less water than usual. When that doesn't work, they may be placed on medication which may give them side effects of dry mouth and blurry vision. Some are helped by topical estrogen, but this is not an option for every person with incontinence. Urethral inserts, pessaries (rigid ring inserted into the vagina), Botox (for overactive bladder), radiofrequency, and sacral nerve stimulators all have had some success. Surgery is an option many women resort to, with mixed results. Some are cured, while some have painful complications.

Among women who have never had children, factors that increase pleasure in the abdomen increase the incidence of UI. Such factors include high BMI, straining due to constipation, high impact exercises, or a high volume of low impact exercises. Sisters of women with UI are at higher risk, as well. In men, Urinary Continence is due to a circular band of muscle that constricts to stop the flow of urine. In contrast, women's continence is supported by several synergistic structures, four of which are easy to grasp: (1) cavernous erectile tissues overlying the first one-third of the urethra; (2) a thin band of muscle overlying but not encircling the cavernous tissues and the first two-thirds of the urethra; (3) the front wall of the vagina and (4) the legs and bulbs of the Clitoris. Once I understood how delicate the female continence mechanism was, I was amazed that it ever worked correctly.

The Clitoris Unveiled

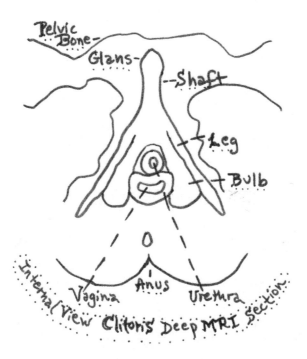

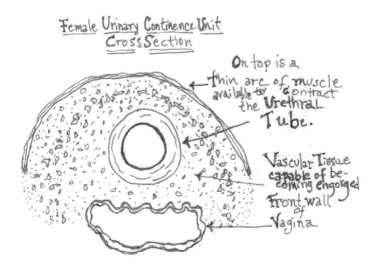

Enlarged Microscopic View

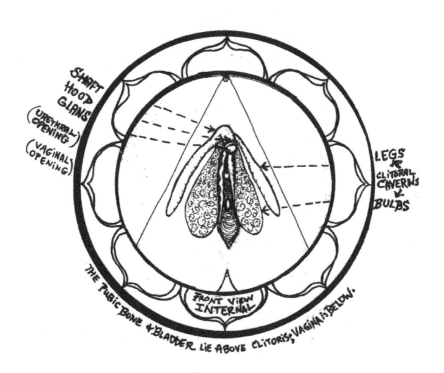

Secrets, Revelations & Research

You can use the following pages for references and notes from your own explorations in unveiling the Clitoris

Owings & Rush

The Clitoris Unveiled

The Clitoris Unveiled

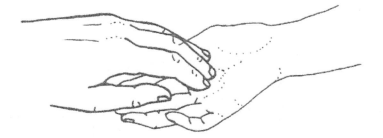

"Most people say that it is the intellect which makes a great scientist. They are wrong: it is character."

Albert Einstein

Owings & Rush

From Emily Porter, M.D., Sexual wellness physician, Austin, Texas:

"Despite graduating from one of the nation's top medical schools, completing gross anatomy, embryology, physiology, and pathology and rotations in obstetrics and gynecology, family medicine, and urology, I don't think we spent a grand total of 30 minutes in 4 years learning about the clitoris. Perhaps that's because, while we study the cause and remedy for erectile dysfunction, there is no such term for women. In fact, anorgasmia in a woman is not considered pathologic unless it causes the woman significant emotional distress and, historically, women are programmed to just accept their fate if they love their partner.

This enlightening book covers everything from the development and anatomy of the clitoris to its male analogue, the penis; the physiology of the organ; and suggestions for how to improve its function. Women need to read this book to understand that the organ they consider their clitoris is really just the tip of the iceberg. Men who realize the importance of the clitoris in orgasm will find it reassuring that their target is substantially larger than they had imagined. And physicians need to read the book because it's time we stop prescribing pills for everything and start opening our ears and listening to our patients. Helping them requires having at least having as much knowledge about the body as they do, a difficult feat in the age of internet education.

I am a sexual wellness physician in Austin, TX and see frustrated women and men daily in my practice. For the women, my training starts with them getting to know what they like and don't like. In order to instruct a lover to please her, a woman must not only know what pleases her, she must also know how to communicate this clearly to him/her. Frustrated husbands, struggling with ED and premature ejaculation, often confide in me that they worry about not being able to please their wives, and when I inquire what they do besides penetration, many are dumbfounded and some don't have any idea that there is a clitoral hood and an entire organ below the tiny nub they can't always easily identify either. Knowing how to please their female partners without penetration tends to take the pressure off them to perform, and often alleviates some of the worry that accompanies their physiologic struggle. When we are enlightened about each other's bodies and our own, there is a comfort with experimentation and a desire to please that most times transcends into a newfound level of sexual gratification.

In addition to reading this wonderful book, I had the pleasure of meeting both the author, Dr. Owings, who truly has a gift for teaching, and Anne Kent Rush, who is as lovely in person as her drawings are in this tribute. I've got a copy of this book on my nightstand and give them freely to my patients in their quest for sexual harmony."

Made in the USA
Monee, IL
09 October 2021